Published By Robert Corbin

@ Lillian Vega

Atkins Diet: Ultimate Atkins Diet's Recipe

Cookbook for Life, Health, and Weight Loss

All Right RESERVED

ISBN 978-1-7385954-4-0

TABLE OF CONTENTS

Spinach Saladgreek Version 1

Cookies With Peanut Butter.. 3

Cheese Scramble 5

Chicken And Pepper Casserole.. 7

Scrambled Eggs, Muffin, Peaches, And Cream Cheese 9

Wild Mushroom Stuffing 12

Irresistible Meatloaf 15

Rockstar Rib Eyesteak... 18

Eggs With Avocado, Salsa And Turkey Bacon Recipe 20

Keto Scotch Eggs Recipe... 22

Chicken With Creamy Bacon Sauce................................ 25

Eggs Benedict With Portobello Mushrooms 28

Ta'ameya (Egyptian Falafel) 30

Rub Noodle Potato Soup.. 32

Chicken Kebabs 34

Sausage Balls 36

Roasted Mixed Vegetables... 38

Mushroom Stuffed Spinach 40

Herbed Asparagus Frittata 42

Roasted Cod With Butter And Garlic Lentil 44

Caulitots 47

Fennel Gratin 49

Asparagus Soup 51

Turkey Club With Watercress And Tomato 53

Cinnamon Churritos 55

Yummy Roast Pork Belly 58

Outstanding Rack Of Lamb 60

Eggs Scrambled With Asparagus, Bacon And Swiss Cheese Recipe 62

Eggs Scrambled With Cheddar, Swiss Chard And Canadian Bacon Recipe 64

Feta Stuffed, Bacon Wrapped Chicken 66

Baconegg Salad Flatout Wrap 68

Fatfree Vegetable Soup 70

Turkey Frame Vegetable Soup 72

Tarragon Tuna 76

Tuna And Egg Salad 78

Cheese Pancake... 80

Green Sandwich 82

Chicken Culets With Mustard.. 83

Salmon Fillet With Cucumber.. 85

Divide Them Into 4 Serving Platters. Sea Bass Fillets With Oat Bran Crust... 87

Chicken Mince Mushrooms... 89

Chicken Greek Salad 91

Eggs And Spinach With Muenster And Pears................. 93

Ham With Green Salad... 95

Phenomenal Herbed Roast Beef 97

Amazing Lamb Chops With Herbed Garlic Sauce........... 99

Vegetarian Black Bean Burgers 102

California Breakfast Burrito Recipe 104

Keto Sausage And Egg Muffin Cups Recipe.................. 107

Baked Chicken With Artichokes 110

Chicken Veggie Soup 113

Chicken And Bok Choy Soup 114

Chicken Avocado Salad 116

Carbless Pork Skewers 118

Sautéed Parsnips 121

Chicken Salad With Avocado 123

Spinach Stuffed Mushrooms 124

Prosciuttowrapped Scallops 127

Tomato Eggs 129

Greek Chicken Herb Salad 131

Avocado Zucchini Soup 134

King Crab Dip 136

Astonishing Chicken Kebabs 138

Keto French Toast Casserole Recipe 140

Eggs Scrambled With Zucchini, Cheddar And Sour Cream Recipe 143

Mushroom Scramble Recipe 144

Noguilt Zesty Ranch Dip 146

Reduced Fat Yogurt Ranch Salad Dressing 148

Sea Bass With Mango Chutney, Ginger, And Black Sesame Seeds 150

Roasted Butterfish... 152

Spinach Salad Greek Version

Ingredients:

- Half red onion, sliced thinly

- 8 ounces of feta cheese, crumbled

- 1 garlic clove, minced

- ¼ cup olive oil

- 3 tbsp red vinegar

- 2 ounces roasted red pepper, drained, cut into strips and patted

- ¼ cup walnut, coarsely chopped

- 1 package of fresh baby spinach, 10 ounce, stemmed, washed and drained

Directions:

1. Take a large bowl and mix vinegar and garlic.
2. Afterward add oil and whisk constantly to become steady and homogenous.
3. Now add spinach along with with onion and mix until coat them.
4. Now mix feta cheese with pepper strips into the mixture and divide them on plate.
5. Sprinkle with chopped walnuts.

Cookies With Peanut Butter

Ingredients:

- Half cup butter, softened
- 1 tsp baking soda
- ¼ tsp salt
- Half cup almond flour
- Half cup ATKINS baking mix
- ¾ cup peanut butter chunky
- Half cup brown sugar twin
- Half cup oat flour
- 2 tsp vital wheat gluten
- Half cup splenda sugar substitute

- 1 large egg

Directions:

1. Blend the sweetener along with eggs and butter and blend until smooth.
2. Add peanut butter afterward and mix well.
3. Add dry Ingredients: and mix properly.
4. Now form balls of the mixture and press them with spoon or fork.
5. Bake them with 375 F for 15 minutes or until browned.

Cheese Scramble

Ingredients:

- Buttery spread (1 ½ tbsp)

- 3 eggs, each of 4 oz [Cholesterol free]

- Black pepper (1/8 tsp), finely crushed

- Basil leaves (½ tsp) [dried and crushed]

- Bread (6 slices) [whole wheat, toasted]

- Cheese (2 tbsp) [low sodium and low fats]

- 1 small red bell pepper, finely chopped

- 1 small sweet onion, finely chopped

Directions:

1. Take a bowl and mix black pepper, eggs and basil together. Set aside.

2. Now melt butter in a medium pan and cook red pepper and onion in it for about 4 minutes until tender.
3. Pout the egg mixture to the pan and let it set for a while.
4. Add cheese over the top and serve.

Chicken And Pepper Casserole

Ingredients:

- Corn flour (2 tsp)//

- 6 thick sliced chestnut mushrooms

- 1 yellow sliced pepper

- ½ large finely chopped onion

- 2 large cubed chicken breast

- A few drops of extra virgin olive oil

- Chicken or vegetable stock (300 mL)

- A sprig of rosemary

- Pepper and salt according to taste

- 1 red pepper, sliced

Directions:

1. Preheat the oven to 180 degrees Celsius.
2. Take chicken in a bowl and add corn flour to coat the chicken.
3. Heat oil in a frying pan over medium high heat and cook onions in it until tender.
4. Add chicken and cook on low until it starts to turn brown.
5. Add mushrooms and pepper and simmer for few minutes more.
6. Now add the chicken stock and let it boil.
7. Take a casserole dish, shift the mixture to the dish and place lid over it.
8. Cook in the preheated oven for about 45 minutes until done.
9. Serve.

Scrambled Eggs, Muffin, Peaches, And Cream Cheese

Ingredients:

- 1 Teaspoon butter

- 1 Teaspoon ground cinnamon

- 1 small tomato

- ½ Hass avocado

- ½ medium peach

- ½ Teaspoon baking powder

- ½ packet granular sugar substitute

- 3 large eggs

- 2 Tablespoons chopped white onion

- 1 Teaspoon olive oil

- 1 Ounce cream cheese

- ¼Cup flax seed meal

Directions:

For the eggs:

1. Cover the nonstick pan with a tablespoon of oil. Heat it on medium high heat.
2. Put it the onions and panfry until translucent.
3. Add in two eggs, together with tomatoes and avocado. Put in the salt and ground black pepper to your taste. Mix them together and cook until the egg is cooked.

For the muffin:

4. Place all the dry Ingredients: together into a coffee mug. Stir them to combine well. Add an

egg and oil or melted butter. Continue stirring.

5. Put into the microwave for about one minute.
6. Topped with cream cheese and serve together with the eggs you cooked and some slices of peach.

Wild Mushroom Stuffing

Ingredients:

- 1 cup chicken broth

- 1 large egg

- 1 teaspoon salt

- ½ cup madeira wine

- ½ cup heavy cream

- ¼ cup chopped fresh parsley

- ¼ teaspoon black pepper

- 9 garlic cloves

- 9 servings Atkins cuisine bread

- 3 tablespoons unsalted butter

- 2 teaspoons fresh thyme

- 2 pounds assorted wild mushrooms

- ¼cup sliced shallots

Directions:

1. Preheat the oven at 170°C. Put butter on baking dish.
2. Melt the butter in a big pan on mediumhigh heat. Put in garlic and shallots; panfry for about 2 minutes.
3. Put in the mushrooms, pepper, and salt; cook for about 8 minutes or until the mushrooms become moisten and the moisture dissolves.
4. Keep cooking for about 6 more minutes or until the liquid evaporates.
5. Turn to heat off. Put the mushroom mixture in a bowl.
6. Add parsley, bread, and thyme, and gently toss in.

7. In another bowl, combine the cream, broth, and egg together; pour in the mushroom mixture and toss to cover it. Transfer the mixture to a baking dish.
8. Bake for about 45 minutes or until it turns golden.

Irresistible Meatloaf

Ingredients:

- 1 tablespoon of hacked thyme

- 1 teaspoon of paprika

- 1 teaspoon of garlic powder

- 1 teaspoon of salt

- 1 teaspoon of dark pepper

- 1 ½ pound of lean ground beef

- 1 beaten egg

- 1 cup of panko breadcrumbs

- 1/3 cup of steak sauce

- 1 finely cleaved onion

- 1 slashed green ringer pepper

- ½ cup of hacked mushrooms

Directions:

1. Preheat your air fryer to 390 degrees Fahrenheit.
2. Using an enormous bowl, add every one of the fixings and mix until it blends properly.
3. Thereafter, oil a hotness safe skillet or the air fryer baking adornment with a nonstick cooking spray.
4. Add the blended ground hamburger into the dish or baking embellishment and straighten the top.
5. After that, place the container or extra inside your air fryer and cook it for 25 minutes at a 390 degrees Fahrenheit or until it gets brown and done.
6. Thereafter, cautiously eliminate it from your air fryer and permit it to chill before serving.

7. Serve and enjoy!

Rockstar Rib Eyesteak

Ingredients:

- 1 teaspoon of sweet paprika
- 1 teaspoon of mustard powder
- 1 teaspoon of onion powder
- 1 teaspoon of stew powder
- 1 teaspoon of garlic powder
- 2 pounds of ribeye steak
- 1 tablespoon of olive oil
- 1 teaspoon of salt
- 1 teaspoon of dark pepper
- 1 teaspoon of ground coriander

- 1 teaspoon of brown sugar

Directions:

1. Preheat your air fryer to 390 degrees Fahrenheit.
2. Sprinkle the olive oil over the ribeye steak. Season the steak on all sides with every one of the recorded flavors until it is well covered.
3. Place the steak into your air fryer basket.
4. Cook it for 8 minutes at a 390 degrees Fahrenheit.
5. After 8 minutes, flip the steak over and cook for 7 extra minutes.
6. When done, cautiously eliminate the steak from your air fryer and permit it to chill before serving.
7. Serve and enjoy!

Eggs With Avocado, Salsa And Turkey Bacon Recipe

Ingredients:

- 1 ounce Salsa

- 2 large Eggs (Whole)

- 2 oz, cookeds Turkey Bacon

- 1/2 fruit without skin and seed California Avocados

Directions:

1. Use the Atkins recipe to make Salsa Cruda or use 2 tablespoons of nosugaradded salsa of your choice.
2. Cook turkey bacon slices on a nonstick skillet over mediumhigh heat until crispy.
3. Slice avocado.

4. Fry eggs (scramble or poach if desired instead).
5. Serve the eggs over sliced avocado topped with salsa and the turkey bacon on the side.

Keto Scotch Eggs Recipe

Ingredients:

- 2 /4 cups Organic High Fiber Coconut Flour

- 12 ounce raw (yield after cooking) Turkey Breakfast Sausage

- 8 large Boiled Eggs

- 1 large Egg (Whole)

- 1 teaspoon Tap Water

Directions:

1. Prepare hardboiled eggs. Cover 8 eggs in a heavy pan with 1inch of cold water.
2. Bring to a rolling boil, remove from the heat and allow eggs to cook for 10 minutes.

3. Immediately drain off hot water and immerse eggs in an icewater bath until cool enough to peel.
4. Peel eggs and dry thoroughly on a paper towel.
5. Whisk 1 egg and water in a small bowl. In another shallow bowl place the coconut flour (season with salt and pepper if desired). Set both aside.
6. Prepare sausage by forming into 8 equal balls.
7. Take each ball and flatten into an oblong disk. Wrap each egg into the sausage disk making sure to cover the entire surface evenly. Set each sausage covered egg on a plate.
8. Heat about 1inch of oil in a large frying pan over mediumhigh heat.
9. Roll each egg in the whisked egg, then the coconut flour until coated all over.

10. When the oil is shimmering, place all 8 eggs (if they fit, allowing at least 1/2inch in between) in the pan.
11. Fry on one side until golden in color then using tongs flip to another side, continue until all sides are golden brown, about 8 minutes total.
12. Drain on a paper towel and serve immediately.

Chicken With Creamy Bacon Sauce

Ingredients:

- 0.36 tsp black pepper

- 4 clove(s) garlic

- 200 ml chicken stock

- 8 bacon

- 2 lemon

- 200 ml double cream

- 3 tbsp olive oil

- 6 chicken thigh

- 0.36 tsp salt

- 3 spring onion

Directions:

1. Heat the oil in a saucepan over medium heat. Season the chicken thighs generously with salt and pepper, makeseason under the skin as well.
2. Add next skinless chicken thighs down in the hot pan.
3. Cook for about 7 minutes, covered with the skin side down, over his shoulder, checking from time to time, until the skin is golden brown.
   Remove chicken from pan.
4. Add minced garlic and a bit 'of chicken broth to soften the pan and cook the garlic for about a minute.
5. Add the remaining chicken broth. Add half of the bacon (cooked, the fat should be drained and cut into small pieces).

6. Add the chicken back to the pan, on top of bacon and the chicken broth.
7. Arrange the lemon slices and thin around the chicken thighs and cook over low heat, covered, for about 30 minutes, until the chicken is done and no longer pink in the center.
8. Once the chicken is cooked, remove from pan. Remove the lemon slices in a pan, it is very important that you remove it now, do not let them in otherwise it will be very bitter sauce.
9. Add the cream to the pan. Bring to a boil and stir, scraping the bottom. Immediately reduce to a boil, add the chicken thighs back into the pan and heat.
10. To serve, spoon some of the sauce over the chicken legs and sprinkle with the remaining chopped bacon and green onion.

Eggs Benedict With Portobello Mushrooms

Ingredients:

- 4 raw egg yolk

- 5 eggs

- 2 tbsp olive oil

- 5 smoked bacon

- 25 tbsp butter

- 4 tbsp lemon juice

- 800 g. portobello mushrooms

Directions:

1. Preheat oven to 200 C.
2. Heat oil in a pan and cook the bacon at will, then continued in the oven to heat.

3. For the sauce, whisk the egg yolks and lemon juice in a sturdy container for the small heat.
4. Place the bowl over a pan of almost boiling water (make sure the touch of sleep bowl of water). Add 2 piece of butter.
5. Stir until melted. Continue to add butter, 2 piece at a time, beating after each addition, until the sauce begins to thicken.
6. When this happens, you can add 45 pieces at a time, continuing until all the butter has been added. If the glass is too hot, remove from heat and continue adding the butter, then return to the pan.
7. If the sauce is too thick, add a little 'hot water. Season with salt and pepper.
8. grilled portobello mushrooms for 6 minutes and put on plates and top with bacon and poached eggs.
9. Spoon over the hollandaise sauce.

Ta'ameya (Egyptian Falafel)

Ingredients:

- ½ cup fresh cilantro
- ½ cup fresh dill
- 3 cloves garlic
- 1 ½ teaspoons ground coriander
- 1 ½ teaspoons salt
- 1 teaspoon ground cumin
- 2 cups dried split fava beans
- 1 red onion, quartered
- ½ cup fresh parsley
- 1 cup sesame seeds (Optional)

- vegetable oil for frying

Directions:

1. Place fava beans in large bowl and cover with several inches of water.
2. Let soak, 8 hours to overnight. Drain.
3. Combine soaked fava beans, red onion, parsley, cilantro, dill, garlic, coriander, salt, and cumin in a food processor; process to a doughlike consistency.
4. Heat a skillet over medium heat. Add sesame seeds; cook, stirring occasionally, until toasted, about 5 minutes. Transfer to a large plate.
5. Shape fava bean mixture into balls. Roll in sesame seeds to coat.
6. Fill a large saucepan 1/4 full with oil; heat over medium heat.
7. Fry fava bean balls in batches until golden brown, 3 to 5 minutes. Drain on paper towels.

Rub Noodle Potato Soup

Ingredients:

- ¼ teaspoon celery salt

- 1 teaspoon salt

- ½ teaspoon ground black pepper

- 1 cup allpurpose flour

- 1 egg

- 4 potatoes, peeled and diced

- 8 cups water to cover

- 1 onion, finely diced

Directions:

1. Place potatoes, onion, water, celery salt, salt, and pepper in Dutch oven and bring to boil.

Reduce heat and let simmer till potatoes are fork tender.
2. Meanwhile, mix rub noodles. Place flour in small bowl, break egg over flour, and mix with fingertips, rubbing mixture together until all flour is absorbed and small lumps form.
3. Drop the dough mixture slowly into boiling potatoes, stirring constantly, and reduce heat.
4. Let simmer 20 minutes, stirring frequently. Add additional salt and pepper to taste.

Chicken Kebabs

Ingredients:

Fat

- 1.5 lbs. chicken tenderloins (approx. 10)

- 1/2 tbsp. rosemary olive oil (or regular)

Other

- 1/2 tbsp. garlic salt

- 1/2 tbsp. lemon pepper seasoning

- 10 6" rosemary skewers (soaked in water for at least 1 hour)

- A few sprigs of fresh thyme

Directions:

1. Preheat oven to 350 degrees.

2. Soak the rosemary skewers for at least 1 hour in water.
3. Use a short sharp knife to twiddle a point on the end of each stick.
4. Toss chicken with Ingredients:. Slide the leaves off the thyme sprigs and sprinkle them in.
5. Skewer the tenderloin with a rosemary stick.
6. Bake at 350 F for 40 minutes.

Sausage Balls

Ingredients:

Fat

- ½ cup of cottage cheese
- 1 egg
- 1 tablespoon butter
- 2 cups of sausages shredded
- ½ cup of cheddar cheese

Other

- 1 teaspoon of chili flakes
- ½ cup of red peppers
- ¼ teaspoon of mustard powder

Directions:

1. Preheat an oven to 350 degrees.
2. Add the egg, chili, and red peppers in a bowl and mix/whisk until the Ingredients: are mixed completely.
3. Mix in the remaining Ingredients:.
4. Using a wooden baking spoon, or cookie scoop, remove the mixture, and handroll the sausage into about two dozen sausage balls.
5. Place the formed balls on a buttered baking pan, or cookie sheet.
6. Bake for about 15 minutes. Serve.
7. You may also store the cooked sausage bags in a covered bowl, or sandwich bags in the refrigerator for later use.

Roasted Mixed Vegetables

Ingredients:

- 2 tablespoons olive oil

- 1/4 large red pepper, diced

- 1/4 large green pepper, diced

- 4 ounces petite carrots

- 1/4 pound whole mushrooms

- 1 medium sized yellow summer squash, peeled, deseeded and cut into small chunks

- 1/4 teaspoon sea salt

- 1/4 teaspoon thyme

- 1/4 teaspoon rosemary

- 1/4 teaspoon onion powder

- 1/4 teaspoon garlic powder

- 1 medium zucchini, cut into small chunks

Directions:

1. Preheat oven to 450 degrees Fahrenheit.
2. Combine the whole mushrooms with the carrots, red and green peppers, yellow squash and zucchini in a roasting pan.
3. Season with salt and add rosemary, onion powder, garlic powder and thyme. Toss well.
4. Bake for 40 minutes. Do not cover. Stir occasionally. Avoid overcooking the vegetables so they don't become mushy.
5. Leftovers should be stored in an airtight container in the fridge. To serve again, reheat on high in the microwave for 2 minutes.

Mushroom Stuffed Spinach

Ingredients:

- 3 crushed garlic cloves

- 1/2 cup parsley, loosely packed

- 1/3 cup white wine vinegar

- 2 teaspoons ground black pepper

- 2 teaspoons kosher salt

- 1 tablespoon olive oil

- 12 ounces sea bass fillet

Directions:

1. Preheat the oven to 450 degrees Fahrenheit.

2. Combine the pepper, salt, and garlic in a cup.
3. Arrange the sea bass fillet on a ceramic baking dish.
4. Rub the garlic mixture on both sides of the fish.
5. Pour wine over the fillet and bake for 15 minutes.
6. After 15 minutes, take it out of the oven and sprinkle with parsley.
7. Place it back to the oven to bake for another 3 minutes.
8. Transfer the fish on a serving plate and pour the remaining juices from the pan over it.

Herbed Asparagus Frittata

Ingredients:

- 1 tbsp dried basil, parsley and oregano
- 1 tbsp butter
- Salt and pepper according to taste
- 6 large eggs
- 6 asparagus spears, chopped
- 2 tbsp chives, chopped

Directions:

1. Preheat the broil and beat eggs in the mixing bowl.
2. Add chives, herb, salt and pepper.
3. Melt butter in oven safe pan and add asparagus.

4. Mix for two to three minutes.
5. Add egg mixture to the pan and mix to distribute them evenly.
6. Cook for 5 minutes over medium high heat until eggs are set and completely done.
7. Place the pan into the oven and broil for 4 minutes until lightly brown.
8. Once finished, removed frittata from pan and cut into servings.
9. Serve this delicious recipe.

Roasted Cod With Butter And Garlic Lentil

Ingredients:

- 1/8 tsp mustard

- 1 tbsp prosciutto, chopped

- 1 tsp almond flour

- 1 tbsp olive oil

- Salt and pepper according to taste

- Lemon wedge for garnish

- 7 ounce of skinless Cof fillet

- 1 tbsp butter, softened

- 1 clove of garlic, finely minced

- 1 tsp lemon juice

Lentils:

- ¼ cup washed lentils

- 1 tbsp butter

- 2 clove minced garlic

- Salt and pepper according to taste

Directions:

1. Take a medium pot and add lentil with ¾ cup of water.
2. Let it boil and soft simmer.
3. Cook for 20 minutes and meanwhile stir salt, pepper, prosciutto, almond flour, mustard, garlic and butter altogether.
4. Preheat oven to 450F.
5. Add oil to the pan over medium high heat, when lentil is done.
6. Seasoning cod fillet with salt and pepper and cook on each side for 4 minutes.

7. Spoon butter over the fillet and bake in the oven for 2 minutes until done completely.
8. Melt butter with high heat and add garlic.
9. Cook until browned, it will take approximately 5 minutes.
10. Add lentil and sauté for 1 minute more.
11. Plate the lentil and topping with cod.
12. Pour sauce over the fish skillet as topping.

Caulitots

Ingredients:

- One 12 ounce bag of frozen cauliflower

- 3 ounce parmesan cheese, grated

- Salt and pepper according to taste

- Garlic powder according to taste

Directions:
1. Preheat oven to 400F.
2. Add cauliflower to microwave for 6 minutes.
3. Discard water and let it cool.
4. Blend them in food processor until smooth.
5. At the same time add parmesan cheese, with salt, pepper and garlic powder in a small bowl.
6. Shape cauliflower in 1.5 inch ball while removing water and add to parmesan cheese mixture.

7. Place the caulitots on baking sheet for 10 minutes before serving.

Fennel Gratin

Ingredients:

- 2 large fennel bulbs, sliced
- Pepper and salt to taste
- Cooking oil
- Oat bran (2 tbsp)
- Low fat cream cheese (2 tbsp)

Directions:

1. Preheat the oven to 180 degrees Celsius.
2. Take fennel bulb in a microwaveable dish and cook in the preheated oven for about 15 minutes.
3. When take out, blend in cream cheese and flavor to taste with pepper and salt.

4. Add oat bran and cooking oil and bake again for about half hour until the oat bran turns to golden brown.
5. Serve.

Asparagus Soup

Ingredients:

- ½ large onion, finely chopped
- Asparagus (400 gm), roughly chopped
- A few drops of extra virgin olive oil
- Vegetable or chicken stock (500 mL)
- A pinch of nutmeg
- Pepper and salt to taste

Directions:
1. Heat olive oil in a frying pan and cook onions in it until translucent.
2. Add asparagus and cook for few more minutes.
3. Now add chicken stock to cover the asparagus completely in it.

4. Cook until the asparagus is done.
5. Remove from the stove and flavor it with pepper and salt.
6. Blend in nutmeg when smooth.
7. Serve and enjoy.

Turkey Club With Watercress And Tomato

Ingredients:

- 2 plum tomatoes

- 1 Pound sliced turkey breast

- 1 Cup chopped watercress leaves

- 1/3 Cup mayonnaise

- 8 Servings Atkins Cuisine Bread

- 8 Pieces crisp cooked bacon

- 2 Tablespoons finely chopped fresh basil

Directions:

1. Fry the bacon in a pan until crispy, put on paper towel and let it absorb the oil.
2. Meanwhile, mix the mayonnaise together with basil.

3. Toast the bread lightly and spread mayonnaise on it.
4. Top four bread slices with the turkey, the watercress, 2 bacon slices, and some tomato slices.
5. Put the remaining slices bread. Cut the sandwich diagonally in two.

Cinnamon Churritos

Ingredients:

- 1 tablespoon unsalted butter

- 1 large egg

- ½ cup flour

- ½ cup unsweetened coconut milk

- ¼ teaspoon baking powder

- 3 tablespoons granular sugar substitute

- 2 tablespoons coconut flour

- 2 teaspoons ground cinnamon

- 1/8 teaspoon salt

Directions:

1. Prepare a pan or deep fryer with 2 up to 3 inches of oil. Preheat at 170°C.
2. Mix the flour, baking powder, coconut flour, cinnamon, and salt together in a bowl. Mix well and set aside.
3. Combine the coconut milk, butter, and a tablespoon of sugar alternative in a small saucepan to a boil.
4. Take out from heat and put in the flour mixture mixing until the texture becomes thick and you can already form balls.
5. Let it be cool for about 5 minutes.
6. When it's already cool, add an egg and mix well until it becomes pastelike texture.
7. Add 4 up to 8 tablespoons of the mixture into the fryer and cook for about 3 minutes or until they become crispy and golden brown.
8. Do it at all the remaining batter. Put on paper towel and let it absorb the oil.

9. Blend a tablespoon of cinnamon with sugar alternative until you get very small granules.
10. Coat the roll with the mixture. Serve and enjoy!

Yummy Roast Pork Belly

Ingredients:

- 1 teaspoon of smoked paprika

- 1 teaspoon of salt

- 2 teaspoons of fivezest powder

- 2 teaspoons of rosemary

- 1 teaspoon of dark pepper

- 2 pounds of pork belly

- 2 teaspoons of garlic powder

- 2 teaspoons of onion powder

Directions:

1. Fill a huge pot with sufficient water, bubble it and afterward add the pork gut into the heated water for 10 minutes.
2. Then eliminate it from the bubbling water and permit it to dry for 3 hours or until it dries completely.
3. Use a fork to punch a few holes by and large around the pork belly.
4. While as yet doing that, utilizing a little blending bowl, gather and blend every one of the flavors into a single unit, then, at that point, rub the pork stomach with the seasonings.

    5. Preheat your air fryer to 320 degrees Fahrenheit.
5. Place the pork paunch inside your air fryer and cook it for 30 minutes.
6. Increase the temperature to 360 degrees Fahrenheit and cook it for 20 extra minutes.

7. Serve and enjoy!

Outstanding Rack Of Lamb

Ingredients:

- 2 tablespoons of olive oil
- 2 tablespoons of honey
- 1 teaspoon of salt
- 1 teaspoon of dark pepper
- 2 racks of lamb
- ¼ cup of newly slashed parsley
- 4 cloves of minced garlic

Directions:

1. Preheat your air fryer to 390 degrees Fahrenheit.

2. Using a blender or food processor, add the parsley, garlic cloves, olive oil, honey, salt, and dark pepper and mix it until it gets absolutely grounded.
3. Rub the grounded parsleygarlic on the sheep racks, without involving them all as you will require them later.
4. Put the barbecue dish frill into your air fryer, and put the sheep racks on top.
5. Cook it for 15 minutes at a 390 degrees Fahrenheit or until it gets brown in color.
6. Spread one more layer of the puree on the sheep racks.
7. Serve and enjoy!

Eggs Scrambled With Asparagus, Bacon And Swiss Cheese Recipe

Ingredients:

- 1 large Egg (Whole)

- 1 ounce Swiss Cheese

- 2 medium slice (yield after cooking) Bacon

- 2 spear, medium (51/4" to 7" long) Asparagus

Directions:

1. Cook bacon in a small skillet over medium high heat.
2. Reserve some of the bacon fat in the skillet and discard the rest or save for another use.
3. Chop bacon into small pieces and set aside.
4. Cook asparagus in skillet with reserved bacon grease until tender, about 3 minutes.
5. Remove and cut into bitesize pieces.

6. Add eggs, bacon, cheese and asparagus back to pan and scramble together until egg is cooked and cheese is melted, about 3 minutes.
7. Or omit the cheese and instead sprinkle over the eggs after they are cooked.
8. Season to taste with salt and freshly ground black pepper.

Eggs Scrambled With Cheddar, Swiss Chard And Canadian Bacon Recipe

Ingredients:

- 2 cups Swiss Chard

- 2 large Eggs (Whole)

- 1/4 cup shredded Cheddar Cheese

- 1 tablespoon Extra Virgin Olive Oil

- 2 ounces CanadianStyle Bacon (Cured)

Directions:

1. Sauté Swiss chard in 1 tsp oil until decreased in volume and tender.
2. Beat eggs slightly and add to pan with Swiss chard. Using a spatula mix to combine and cook till eggs are set.

3. Add shredded Cheddar cheese and Canadian bacon to top or it may be added in with the eggs and cooked all together.

Feta Stuffed, Bacon Wrapped Chicken

Ingredients:

- 200 g. fresh baby spinach

- 80 g. feta cheese

- 6 tbsp cream cheese

- 3 clove(s) garlic

- 500 g. chicken breast, raw, skinless

- 8 bacon

Directions:

1. In a nonstick place spinach and cook, stirring for a few minutes until the leaves dry. Allow to cool.
2. Squeezing water spinach and use a knife to cut spinach or less.

3. Add this in a bowl with the chopped garlic, cream cheese and feta cheese.
4. Stir until well combined. With a sharp knife cut a small opening in the side of each chicken breast.
5. The relatively narrow gap maintenance expand the domestic cut to form a bag.
6. With a teaspoon, scoop the mixture of spinach and cheese in space, filling as much as possible.
7. Take two slices of bacon for the chicken breast and wrap around the breast to seal the opening is cut, and keep the fill.
8. Heat oil in a large skillet over medium heat.
9. Add the chicken once the pan is hot, cook for about 68 minutes per side or until golden brown on the outside and cooked all the way.

Baconegg Salad Flatout Wrap

Ingredients:

- 2/3 tsp or 2 packet yellow mustard

- 2 flatbread light original flatbread

- 2 2/3 oz, cookeds turkey bacon

- 3 large boiled eggs

- 2 tbsp real mayonnaise

- 2 inner leaf romaine lettuce (salad)

Directions:

1. Mix together the chopped eggs, mayonnaise and mustard.
2. Add salt and pepper to taste.
   mixture of diffusion in a rounded end having the lettuce flattened Flatout on it.

3. Top with crumbled bacon cooked and then wrapped and cut in half.

Fatfree Vegetable Soup

Ingredients:

- 2 green bell peppers, diced

- 1 (28 ounce) can whole peeled tomatoes with liquid, mashed

- 1 tablespoon chicken bouillon powder

- ¼ teaspoon ground black pepper

- 2 teaspoons curry powder (Optional)

- 3 cups finely shredded cabbage

- 2 stalks celery, chopped

- 1 ½ cups cauliflower florets

- 14 cups water

- 2 onions, chopped

- 2 large carrots, sliced

- 2 potatoes, peeled and cubed

- 3 teaspoons dried dill weed

Directions:
1. In a large cooking pot, measure water, add onions, carrots, potatoes, green peppers, mashed tomatoes, chicken bouillon powder, black pepper, and curry powder.
2. Boil for 20 minutes or until carrots are tender.
3. Add shredded cabbage, chopped celery, cauliflower florets, and dill weed, and cook an additional 10 to 15 minutes.
4. If soup is too thick, add more water and bring to boil. Adjust seasonings to taste.

Turkey Frame Vegetable Soup

Ingredients:

- 8 cups water

- water to cover

- 1 turnip, peeled and cubed

- 2 parsnips, peeled and sliced

- 3 carrots, chopped

- ½ cup frozen green beans

- ½ cup frozen green peas

- 1 (15 ounce) can red beans, drained and rinsed

- ¼ cup chopped fresh parsley

- 1 turkey carcass

- 2 carrots, chopped

- 2 stalks celery, cut into 2 inch pieces

- 1 onions, chopped

- 4 cloves garlic, minced

- 4 sprigs fresh parsley

- 12 black peppercorns

- 2 bay leaves

- 1 teaspoon dried thyme

- 1 tablespoon chicken bouillon granules

Directions:

1. Place turkey carcass in a large pot over high heat.

2. Add the carrots, celery, onion, garlic, parsley sprigs, peppercorns, bay leaves, thyme, chicken bouillon granules, water and enough water to cover all.
3. Bring to a boil, uncovered, then reduce heat to medium low and let simmer for 1 1/2 hours.
4. Remove the turkey carcass and allow it to cool.
5. Remove any meat from the carcass, cut into bitesized pieces and set aside. Strain the stock through a sieve OR a colander covered with cheesecloth into another large pot.
6. Discard the unstrained iINGREDIENTS:. Place the turkey meat into the pot, cover and refrigerate overnight.
7. The next day, use a slotted spoon to remove the fat that has solidified on top of the stock.

8. Return the stock to a large pot over high heat, add the turnip, parsnips and carrots and bring to a boil.
9. Reduce heat to low, cover and simmer for one hour, or until vegetables are tender.
10. Add the green beans, peas and beans and allow to heat through, about 15 minutes.
11. Finally add the chopped parsley and season with salt and pepper to taste.

Tarragon Tuna

Ingredients:

Fat:

- 2 teaspoons mayonnaise
- 1 teaspoon olive oil
- Two 6ounce tuna steaks, 1 inch thick

Other:

- 2 tablespoons minced fresh or 2 teaspoons dried tarragon plus tarragon sprigs for garnish
- Salt and cracked pepper to taste

Directions:

1. Stir together the mayo and tarragon in a small bowl. Cover and set aside.
2. Heat a heavy skillet or ridged grill pan over mediumhigh heat.

3. Pat the tuna dry with paper towels, then season to taste with salt and cracked pepper.
4. Dab olive oil over the surfaces of the fish.
5. Pan grilled the fish for about 3 minutes per side for medium. Transfer to warmed dinner plates.
6. Top each steak with a dollop of tarragon mayonnaise, and garnish with tarragon sprigs.
7. Place a mound of squash beside the tuna.

Tuna And Egg Salad

Ingredients:

Fat

- 2 (6ounce) cans tuna (try to get those packed in oil
- 1/2 cup mayonnaise
- 2 large hardboiled eggs

Other

- 11/2 teaspoon salt
- 1/2 teaspoon black pepper
- /4 cup diced white onion
- 1/4 cup sugarfree relish

Directions:

1. Put eggs in a medium mixing bowl and mash with a fork.
2. Add tuna and mayonnaise and mash together until Ingredients: are combined.
3. Stir in onion, relish, salt, and pepper.

Cheese Pancake

Ingredients:

- 1 packet Stevia
- 4 ounces cream cheese
- 2 eggs
- 1 tablespoon ground flax seed
- 1/2 teaspoon ground cinnamon

Directions:

1. Beat the egg whites in a small bowl.
2. On a separate bowl, beat the cream cheese with an electric mixer until smooth.
3. Combine the egg yolk with the cream cheese. Add the flax seed, salt, Stevia and cinnamon. Continue to beat the mixture.
4. Fold in the beaten egg whites.

5. Put a pan over medium heat and add a small amount of butter.
6. Scoop 1/4 cup from the mixture.
7. Cook the pancake for 2 to 3 minutes or until golden brown. Then, serve.

Green Sandwich

Ingredients:

- 70 grams chopped spinach
- 1 ounce cream cheese
- 1 teaspoon finely chopped garlic
- 1 egg
- Salt and pepper

Directions:
1. Preheat oven to 180 degrees Fahrenheit.
2. Beat the egg in a bowl.
3. Stir in chopped garlic and spinach.
4. Season with salt and pepper. Whisk well.
5. Pour the mixture into a baking tin. Put inside the oven to bake for 10 to 15 minutes.

6. Set it aside to cool. Cut into pieces and serve with cream cheese on top.

Chicken Culets With Mustard

Ingredients:

- ¾ tsp crashed black pepper

- 1 egg

- 8 ounce chicken culets

- 1 scallion, chopped

- Half cup all purpose ATKINS mix

- 1 tsp salt

- 2 tbsp heavy cream

- 6 tbsp extra virgin olive oil

- 1 ½ tbsp mustard

Directions:

1. Add salt, pepper and baking mix in a deep pot.
2. Take a separate bowl and beat eggs with heavy cream.
3. Dip chicken culets in egg and then in the baking sheet.
4. Take a pan and heat olive oil over medium high heat.
5. Cook cutlets until golden brown and keep them aside.
6. Discard oil from the pan to another pot and add heavy cream.
7. Let it boil, then add scallion and cook until thickens.
8. Remove from heat and add salt, mustard and pepper.

Salmon Fillet With Cucumber

Ingredients:

- 1 tbsp olive oil

- 2 tsp rice vinegar

- Half tsp salt

- 2 tbsp unsalted butter

- Salmon fillets

- 1 tsp fresh tarragon, finely chopped

- 2 small cucumber, seedless

- ¼ tsp black pepper

- Half tsp granular sugar substitute

Directions:

1. Add pepper, salt and cucumber slices to the bowl.
2. Take a pan and heat butter and oil in it.
3. Seasoning fish and cook for 4 minutes on each side.
4. Place the paper towel on top to absorb excess oil.
5. Add remaining butter and add cucumber.
6. Add vinegar, sugar and tarragon.

Divide Them Into 4 Serving Platters. Sea Bass Fillets With Oat Bran Crust

Ingredients:

- Ground black pepper to taste
- Water (2 tbsp)
- A handful of finely chopped fresh flat leaf parsley
- 4 sea bass fillets
- Extra virgin olive oil for spraying
- The leaves of few sprigs of fresh thyme
- Oat bran (4 tbsp)

Directions:

1. Preheat the oven to 180 degrees Celsius.

2. Prepare the breadcrumbs by mixing water, herbs and oat bran in a bowl.
3. The oat bran will absorb the water and give a look of coarse breadcrumbs.
4. Take a baking tray and place the fillets without skin in it and daub a layer of breadcrumbs on each fillet.
5. Spray the fillets with oil and cook in the preheated oven for about 1012 minutes until the breadcrumbs turns to brown.
6. Serve.

Chicken Mince Mushrooms

Ingredients:

- Salt (1 tsp)

- Extra virgin olive oil (1 tbsp)

- Chilli con carne spice mix (1 packet)

- 8 chestnuts mushrooms, quartered

- ½ red onion, chopped

- Chicken (600 gm), minced

- Low fat natural yogurt (4 tbsp)

- Boiling water (125 mL)

- Canned tomatoes (800 gm), chopped

Directions:

1. Preheat the oven to 180 degrees Celsius.

2. Mix all the Ingredients: in a bowl and shift to the microwaveable casserole dish.
3. Cover the dish and cook in the preheated oven for about 90 minutes. Stir occasionally.
4. Add low fat yogurt to each portion and serve.

Chicken Greek Salad

Ingredients:

- 1 little gem lettuce

- ½ red pepper, diced

- Cooked chicken (300 gm)

- 1 peeled and diced cucumber

- ½ small red onion, finely sliced

- Olive oil for spray

- Dried oregano (1 tbsp)

- 3 medium size tomatoes, diced

Directions:

1. Combine all the Ingredients: together in a medium size bowl and spray with cooking spray.
2. Serve and enjoy. Serve with cucumber as topping.

Eggs And Spinach With Muenster And Pears

Ingredients:

- 1 ounceweight muenster cheese

- 1 teaspoon extravirgin olive oil

- 1 medium pear

- 2 cups chopped spinach

- 2 large eggs

Directions:

1. Put the spinach in a hot pan with a tablespoon of oil. Cook until floppy.
2. Break the eggs on pan with spinach and mix them together while the heat is on until cooked.
3. You can add salt and pepper to taste.

4. Serve the eggs with Muenster cheese and slices of pear.

Ham With Green Salad

Ingredients:

- 1 medium carrot

- ½ cup chopped jicama

- ½ large green bell pepper

- ¼ cup canned chickpeas

- ¼ cup frozen corn

- 6 ounces ham

- 2 cups mixed greens

- 1 serving creamy Italian dressing

Directions:

1. Use the recipe from Atkins recipe in order to make Creamy Italian Dressing for the salad.

2. Mix all the Ingredients: and toss together with the dressing. Enjoy!

Phenomenal Herbed Roast Beef

Ingredients:

- 1 teaspoon of dark pepper

- 1 teaspoon of dried thyme

- 1 tablespoon of newly slashed rosemary

- 1 tablespoon of newly cleaved parsley

- 4pound simmered beef

- 1 tablespoon of olive oil

- 1 teaspoon of salt

Directions:

1. Preheat your air fryer to 360 degrees Fahrenheit.

2. Using a bowl, add and blend the olive oil, salt, dark pepper, thyme, rosemary, parsley properly.
3. Rub the combination all around the broiled beef.
4. Place the meat inside your air fryer bin and cook it for 20 minutes.
5. After 20 minutes, flip the hamburger over and cook for 30 extra minutes or until it comes to your ideal preference.
6. Remove the broiled hamburger and permit it to cool of before serving.
7. Serve and enjoy!

Amazing Lamb Chops With Herbed Garlic Sauce

Ingredients:

- 1 tablespoon of newly cleaved parsley
- 1 tablespoon of newly slashed oregano
- 2 tablespoons of olive oil
- 1 teaspoon of onion powder
- 1 teaspoon of salt
- 4 sheep chops
- 1 garlic bulb
- 1 teaspoon of dark pepper

Directions:

1. Preheat your air fryer to 390 degrees Fahrenheit.
2. Brush the garlic bulb with an olive oil and spot it inside your air fryer,cook it for 12 minutes or until it is appropriately cooked, then, at that point, eliminate it from your air fryer and set it aside.
3. Using a little bowl, blend the parsley, oregano, olive oil, onion powder, salt, and the dark pepper properly.
4. Thereafter spread each sheep hack with around one teaspoon of the herbed olive oil mixture.
5. Place the sheep cleaves into your air fryer and cook it for 6 minutes at a 390 degrees Fahrenheit or until it becomes brown.
6. Press the garlic cloves with a garlic press and blend it appropriately with the herbed olive oil.

7. Spread the garlic sauce over the sheep chops.
8. Serve and enjoy!

Vegetarian Black Bean Burgers

Ingredients:

- 1 Jalapeno Pepper

- 1/3 cup Flax Seed Meal

- 1 1/2 teaspoons Chili Powder

- 1/2 teaspoon Salt

- 1/2 teaspoon Black Pepper

- 8 teaspoons Olive Oil

- 15 ounces Black Beans (Canned)

- 1 small whole (22/5" diameter) Tomato

- 1/4 cup Cilantro

- 1 large Egg

Directions:

1. Preheat oven to 375°F.
2. Place 1 teaspoon of oil in 4 spots on a rimmed baking sheet evenly spaced for four 4inch burgers.
3. Drain and rinse black beans then mash with a fork leaving some intact.
4. Add the diced tomatoes, chopped cilantro, diced jalapeno, flax meal, chili powder, salt and pepper.
5. Mix to blend then add the egg and blend until thoroughly combined.
6. Using a 1/3 cup measure, place 4 equal sized burgers onto the baking sheet and flatten slightly till about 1/2inch thick.
7. Sprinkle with 1 teaspoon of oil each and bake covered with aluminum foil for 30 minutes then uncover and bake an additional 10 minutes until fully set.

8. Remove from the oven and allow to rest for 10 minutes before plating.

California Breakfast Burrito Recipe

Ingredients:

- 1/2 teaspoon Salt

- 1/4 teaspoon Black Pepper

- 8 large Eggs (Whole)

- 1/8 teaspoon Red or Cayenne Pepper

- 9 sprigs Cilantro (Coriander)

- 1/2 cup shredded Cheddar Cheese

- 4 tortillas Low Carb Tortillas

- 1 tablespoon Canola Vegetable Oil

- 3 large Scallions or Spring Onions

- 4 ounces Green Chili Peppers (Canned)

- 1 medium whole (23/5" diameter) Red Tomato

Directions:
1. Use 1/4 cup total of the Atkins recipe for Tomatillo Salsa.
2. Heat oven to 325° F.
3. Wrap tortillas in foil and heat in oven 510 minutes.
4. In a medium nonstick skillet, heat oil over mediumhigh heat.
5. Dice the green onions, chiles, and tomatos.
6. Add them to the pan and season with salt and pepper. Sauté for 3 minutes.
7. Push mixture to side of pan. Add eggs and cayenne to skillet.
8. Cook, 12 minutes, stirring occasionally with rubber spatula, until soft, creamy curds form.
9. Stir vegetable mixture into eggs.

10. Divide mixture among warm tortillas, sprinkle with cilantro, one tablespoon of salsa and 2 tablespoons cheese. Roll up tortillas.

15.

Keto Sausage And Egg Muffin Cups Recipe

Ingredients:

- 1/4 teaspoon Paprika

- 1/8 teaspoon Nutmeg (Ground)

- 1/2 teaspoon Salt

- 1/4 teaspoon Black Pepper

- 2/3 cup chopped Sweet Red Peppers

- 13 large Eggs (Whole)

- 12 ounces Pork Italian Sausage

- 2/3 pound Ground Turkey

- 1/4 teaspoon leaf Dried Thyme Leaves

- 1 tablespoon Parsley (Dried)

- 1/8 teaspoon Red or Cayenne Pepper

Directions:

1. Preheat oven to 350°F. Grease a muffin tin with twelve wells.
2. Combine the sausage and ground turkey until thoroughly mixed.
3. Add thyme, parsley, cayenne, paprika, nutmeg, salt, black pepper, chopped red bell peppers and 1 egg.
4. Mix together with hands until all iINGREDIENTS: are incorporated.
5. Divide sausage mixture evenly between the 12 muffin wells.
6. Push mixture up and slightly over the rims of the wells making sure there are no holes.
7. Crack an egg into each well and immediately place in oven. Bake for 2530 minutes until eggs are set.

8. Top with cheese and hot sauce or salsa if desired (don't forget to add the extra grams of NC if you do).

Baked Chicken With Artichokes

Ingredients:

- 2/3 tsp black pepper

- 4 tablespoons extra virgin olive oil

- 2/3 cup, chopped onions

- 8 oz mushroom pieces and stems

- 5 2/3 tsps garlic

- 2 package (9 oz), yield artichokes (globe or french) (with salt, frozen, drained, cooked, boiled)

- 2 tsp rosemary

- 2/5 tsp crushed red pepper flakes

- 5 fl oz sauvignon blanc wine

- 30 oz, boneless, raw (yield after cooking)

- Chicken thigh

- 2/3 tsp salt

- 2 2/3 tsp, grounds oregano

- 4/5 serving atkins flour mix

Directions:

1. Use the recipe for Atkins Atkins combine flour for this recipe.
2. Dredge chicken in flour before browning seals in juices and give it a nice color.
   Preheat oven to 460 F baking mix 2/5 cup salt and pepper in a flat dish and mix well. dredge chicken mixture, turning to evenly coat and then beating to remove any excess.
3. In a large pot, heat the oil over mediumhigh heat.

4. Bake until lightly browned chicken, turning once, about 5 minutes. Transfer to a baking sheet.
5. Add the chopped onion to the pan and saute until soft, about 3 minutes.
6. Add the sliced mushrooms and saute saute about 4 minutes ,.
7. Add the minced garlic and stirfry until the aroma is released about 40 seconds.
8. Add the wine, artichokes, rosemary and red pepper flakes and bring to a boil.
9. Pour the mixture over the chicken artichoke in a pan, cover and cook 50 minutes, until the chicken is cooked and tender.
10. Add salt and pepper also, if desired, and stirred under the oregano before serving.

Chicken Veggie Soup

Ingredients:

- 2 potatoes, peeled and cubed

- ½ (4.5 ounce) can mushrooms, drained

- 2 (14.5 ounce) cans chicken broth

- 1 cup baby carrots, halved

Directions:

1. In a large saucepan over medium high heat, combine the chicken stock, carrots and potatoes and simmer for 20 minutes, or until potatoes are tender.
2. Add the mushrooms and simmer for 5 more minutes.

Chicken And Bok Choy Soup

Ingredients:

- 4 teaspoons chicken soup base (such as Better than Bouillon®)

- 6 small potatoes, diced

- 4 carrots, sliced

- 6 large bok choy ribs with leaves, finely chopped

- 2 stalks celery, sliced

- 2 skinless, boneless chicken breast halves, cut into 1/2inch cubes

- 1 tablespoon vegetable oil

- 1 yellow onion, diced

- 2 cloves garlic, minced

- 6 cups water

Directions:

1. Heat vegetable oil in a large stockpot over medium heat; cook and stir onion and garlic in the hot oil until onion is softened and translucent, about 10 minutes.
2. Add water, chicken base, potatoes, carrots, bok choy, and celery; bring to a boil. Reduce heat and simmer until vegetables are slightly tender, about 10 minutes.
3. Add chicken; continue simmering until chicken is no longer pink in the center, about 10 minutes.

Chicken Avocado Salad

Ingredients:

Fat

- 1 teaspoon olive oil

- 1 medium avocado, cubed

- 1 (12.5ounce) can shredded chicken breast

- 1/2 cup Homemade Mayonnaise

Other

- 1/2 teaspoon black pepper

- 1/4 teaspoon paprika

- 1 teaspoon fresh lemon juice

- 2 tablespoons sliced black olives

- 1/2 teaspoon garlic salt

Directions:

1. Put all Ingredients: in a medium mixing bowl and mash with a fork until combined.

Carbless Pork Skewers

Ingredients:

Fat

- 2 lbs. pork shoulder
- 1 cup virgin olive oil (may be reused later on)

Other

- 4 tbsp. freshly chopped oregano
- 2 tsp. sea salt
- Dash of freshly ground black pepper
- 4 wooden or stainless steel skewers
- Juice from 2 large lemons
- 2 tbsp. balsamic vinegar
- 4 tbsp. freshly chopped mint

Directions:

1. To prepare the marinade, rinse the mint and oregano and drain thoroughly.
2. Chop the herbs and preserve these apart in a small bowl.
3. Cube the pork into big cubes. Place them in a medium bowl and pour the olive oil on them.
4. Add the chopped herbs and season with balsamic vinegar.
5. Season with salt and freshly grounded black pepper to taste.
6. Combine all the Ingredients:, and ensure the meat is submerged in oil. Let it relax in the fridge for 8 to 12 hours.
7. When the meat is marinated, use the grill to preheat the oven to 450 degrees.
8. Note that the meat will barely change color after you take it out from the fridge. This is fine.

9. Skewer the meat pieces in four skewer sticks. Place them on a rack and within the oven.
10. After about 10 minutes, flip the skewers, and cook until done.

Sautéed Parsnips

Ingredients:

- 1/4 tablespoon butter

- 1 medium parsnip

- 1 pinch salt and pepper

Directions:

1. Remove the ends of the parsnips, peel and cut them into rings.
2. Wash and place them in a microwave safe dish with 1/8 cup of water.
3. Heat on high in the microwave for 5 to 7 minutes.
4. Heat a nonstick pan and melt the butter over medium heat.
5. Drain the parsnips and add to the pan.

6. Cook each side for a few minutes until they turn light brown.
7. Sprinkle with salt and pepper then, serve.

Chicken Salad With Avocado

Ingredients:

- 1 tablespoon chopped cilantro

- 1/2 avocado cut in cubes

- 1 cup poached chicken, cut in cubes

- 4 Bib lettuce leaves

- 1 small pinch salt

- 1 teaspoon lime juice

Directions:

1. Combine the avocado, chicken, lime, cilantro and salt in a mixing bowl.
2. Lay the lettuce leaves flat on a serving plate.
3. Scoop the salad mixture and place over the lettuce.

Spinach Stuffed Mushrooms

Ingredients:

- 8 mushrooms with stems removed

- TofuSpinach filling

- ¼ cup onion, diced

- 7 ounce tofu firm, drained and crumbled

- 2 tbsp tahini

- 2 tbsp basil

- ¼ tsp black pepper, grounded

- 2 tbsp lemon juice

- 1 tbsp tamari

- 2 tbsp water

- 1 tsp tamari

- 1 tbsp virgin olive oil

- 2 medium garlic, finely minced

- 2 tbsp nutritional yeast

- ¼ cup spinach, chopped

- Half tsp salt

- Red pepper flakes

- 1 tsp tamari

Directions:
1. Mix water, tamari and lemon juice altogether in a dish.
2. Add mushrooms and soak while preparing filling.
3. Take a small pan and add olive oil.
4. Cook garlic and onion for 3 minutes.

5. Now add tofu and stir instantly for a while.
6. Add spinach, black pepper, basil, tamari, salt and red bell pepper and mix it well.
7. Remove from heat and scoop filling with mushrooms caps.
8. Bake for 15 minutes before serving.

Prosciuttowrapped Scallops

Ingredients:

- 3 ounce of extra virgin oil

- 2 tbsp of vinegar

- 8 pieces of prosciutto

- 2 cups of radicchio

- 1 Shallot

- Salt and pepper according to taste

- 8 large sea scallops

- 2 cups Belgian evdive

- 1 tomato plum

Directions:

1. Preheat oven to 400 F and cut tomatoes, shallot in a bowl with olive oil.
2. Add pepper and salt according to taste.
3. Now add tomato and shallot to the baking sheet until lightly browned.
4. Set them aside and blend tomatoes, shallots and vinegar together.
5. Seasoning it with salt and pepper.
6. Add olive oil for emulsification.
7. Cover each scallop with prosciutto.
8. Heat the pan and add the remaining oil.
9. Cook scallops until done then keep it aside.
10. Add radicchio and endive to the pan and mix for 5 minutes instantly.
11. Add the roasted tomato mixture.
12. Add radicchio mixture on each plate and add scallop as topping.

Tomato Eggs

Ingredients:

- Warm water (3 tbsp)
- ½ large onion, chopped
- Vegetable oil for spray
- 4 eggs
- A few roughly chopped leaves of fresh basil
- Chopped tomatoes (400 gm)
- Pepper and salt to taste

Directions:
1. Take a nonstick frying pan, spray with oil and heat over medium high heat.
2. Cook onion in it for few minutes until tender.

3. Add tomatoes and 3 tablespoons of water and mix well.
4. Cook for about 1015 minutes but if it is too thick then add little water.
5. Put in basil and mix until the tomatoes absorb basil.
6. Break and pour the egg over the mixture and flavor it with pepper and salt.
7. Serve when the eggs are done.

Greek Chicken Herb Salad

Ingredients:

- Grape tomatoes (1 cup), cut into halves

- English cucumber (1 cup), peeled and chopped

- Romaine lettuce (8 cups), finely chopped

- Minced garlic (1 tsp), bottled

- Fatfree plain yogurt (1 cup)

- Tahini sesame seed pasta (2 tsp)

- Lemon juice (5 tsp)

- Cheese (¼ cup), crumbled

- 6 kalamata olives (cut into half and pits removed)

- Skinless and boneless chicken breast (1 pound), slice into cubes

- Cooking spray

- Dried oregano (1 tsp)

- Salt (½ tsp), divided equally

- Garlic (½ tsp), finely crashed

- Black pepper (¾ tsp), divided equally

Directions:
1. Mix garlic powder, ¼ tsp oregano, ¼ tsp salt and ½ tsp pepper together in a bowl.
2. Take a non sticky pan spray with cooking oil and heat over medium high heat.
3. Add chicken and spices mixture and cook thoroughly.
4. Splash with lemon juice and then take out.

5. Now mix salt, pepper, juice, yogurt, sesame seed paste and garlic together in a separate bowl and stir gently.
6. Toss with olives, cucumber, lettuce and tomatoes and shift the mixture to the serving plates.
7. Place half cup of chicken mixture over each one, splash with cheese and drizzle with yogurt.
8. Serve and enjoy the delicious recipe.

Avocado Zucchini Soup

Ingredients:

- 2 medium zucchini

- 1 teaspoon ginger root

- 1 garlic clove

- 1 tablespoon lemon juice

- 1 Hass avocado

- 1 tablespoon chopped red bell pepper

- 1 cup water

- 29 fluid ounces vegetable broth

- 4 green onions

- 2 tablespoons extravirgin olive oil

- ½ teaspoon salt

- ¼ teaspoon pepper

Directions:

1. Heat the oil in a saucepan on medium heat.
2. Add 2/3 of green onions and cook for about 3 minutes; combine the garlic and ginger together and cook for one more minute.
3. Add water, broth, salt, zucchini, and pepper.
4. Cover and let it cook for 10 minutes or until the zucchini gets soft. Stir the avocado after it's cooked.
5. Pound soup in the food processor or blender.
6. Put back into pan to heat through and mix together with lemon juice.
7. Finish off by serving it together with red pepper and green onions.

King Crab Dip

Ingredients:

- 2 tablespoons finely chopped green bell pepper
- 1 tablespoon fresh dill
- ½ teaspoon garlic powder
- ½ cup finely chopped red bell pepper
- 3/4 cup cooked king crab meat
- 2 ounces cream cheese, softened
- 2 teaspoons fresh lemon juice
- 2 tablespoons mayonnaise
- 2 green onions

Directions:

1. Mix mayonnaise, cream cheese, garlic powder, and lemon juice until smooth.
2. Combine the peppers, crab meat, dill, and green onion.
3. Put some Tabasco to taste.
4. Chill for about an hour to let the flavors to blend. Serve.

Astonishing Chicken Kebabs

Ingredients:

- 1/3 cup of honey

- 1/3 cup of soy sauce

- 1 teaspoon of salt

- 1 teaspoon of dark pepper

- Wooden skewers

- 2 slashed boneless, skinless chicken breasts

- 6 parts of mushrooms

- 1 cleaved red chime pepper

- 1 slashed green ringer pepper

- 1 slashed yellow ringer pepper

Directions:

1. Preheat your air fryer to 340 degrees Fahrenheit.
2. Using a bowl, add and blend 1/3 cup of honey, 1/3 cup of soy sauce, salt, and dark pepper.
3. For each wooden stick, add the ringer peppers, chicken, and mushroom slices.
4. Thereafter, brush the chicken kabobs with the honey soy sauce mixture.
5. Place the chicken kabobs into your air fryer bin and cook it for 15 to 20 minutes.
6. Serve and enjoy!

Keto French Toast Casserole Recipe

Ingredients:

- 3/4 teaspoon Salt

- 1 cup Heavy Cream

- 1 cup Coconut Milk Unsweetened

- 1 teaspoon Cinnamon

- 1/4 teaspoon Nutmeg (Ground)

- 1/2 cup Sugar Free Maple Flavored Syrup

- 14 large Eggs (Whole)

- 3 tablespoons Xylitol

- 10 tablespoons Unsalted Butter Stick

- 1 cup Organic High Fiber Coconut Flour

- 1 1/2 teaspoons Baking Powder (Straight Phosphate, Double Acting)

Directions:

1. It is best but not necessary to make the bread portion of this recipe a day or more ahead (a week in advance works great).
2. Preheat oven to 350°F. Grease a small bread pan (8x4inches). Set aside.
3. Whisk together 8 eggs, 1 tablespoon xylitol and melted butter in a medium bowl.
4. Sift together the coconut flour, baking powder and 3/4 teaspoon salt. Add to the egg mixture and blend until thickened. Bake for 3540 minutes until the sides pull away from the pan and are golden brown. Allow to cool in the pan for 10 minutes then transfer to a wire rack to finish cooling; about 30 minutes. If baking in advance, once cool, place in an airtight container or zip top bag and refrigerate for up to 2 weeks. If using

immediately, once cool, break into 1inch pieces and place in the same pan used to bake the bread or a small casserole dish.

5. In a medium bowl, whisk together 6 eggs, heavy cream, coconut milk (soy milk or water can replace the coconut milk), 2 tablespoons xylitol, cinnamon, nutmeg and a pinch of salt. Pour over bread and bake for 50 minutes at 350°F until it is set in the center. Serve immediately by dividing into 8 servings and drizzle each serving with 2 teaspoons sugarfree pancake syrup (or about 1/3 cup over the whole casserole).

Eggs Scrambled With Zucchini, Cheddar And Sour Cream Recipe

Ingredients:

- 1 teaspoon extra virgin olive oil

- 1/2 cup chopped zucchini

- 1/4 cup shredded cheddar cheese

- 2 large eggs (whole)

- 2 tablespoons sour cream (cultured)

Directions:
1. Lightly beat together eggs and sour cream. Set aside.
2. Heat a skillet over mediumhigh heat. Lightly sauté zucchini in oil for 2 minutes.

3. Add eggsour cream mixture and cheese to the skillet and scramble together until thoroughly cooked.

Mushroom Scramble Recipe

Ingredients:

- 14 ounces firm silken tofu

- 1 cup baby spinach

- 1/4 cup shredded cheddar cheese

- 3 tablespoons parmesan cheese (grated)

- 4 large eggs (whole)

- 1/8 teaspoon leaf dried thyme leaves

- 1 cup mushroom pieces and stems

- 1/2 cup chopped onions

- 3 tablespoons extra virgin olive oil

- 8 cherry tomatoes

Directions:

1. In a large nonstick skillet, over mediumhigh heat, cook the white onion and mushrooms in the oil until soft (about 3 minutes).
2. Add the tofu and spinach and cook an additional 3 minutes.
3. Stir in the tomatoes, eggs, Cheddar and Parmesan cheeses and 1/8 tsp thyme and cook until the egg is firm.

Noguilt Zesty Ranch Dip

Ingredients:

- 1 teaspoon garlic powder
- 1 teaspoon onion powder
- 1 teaspoon prepared horseradish, or to taste
- ½ teaspoon dried basil
- ½ teaspoon dried thyme
- ½ teaspoon ground black pepper, or to taste
- ¼ teaspoon paprika
- ¼ teaspoon chili powder
- ¼ teaspoon sea salt
- ¼ teaspoon dried dill weed

- 1 cup fatfree plain yogurt

- ½ cup reducedfat mayonnaise

- ½ cup fatfree sour cream

- 4 green onions, chopped

- 3 tablespoons bacon bits

- 1 tablespoon dried parsley

Directions:
1. Place the yogurt, mayonnaise, sour cream, green onions, and bacon bits in a mixing bowl.
2. Season with parsley, garlic powder, onion powder, horseradish, basil, thyme, pepper, paprika, chili powder, sea salt, and dill. Mix until evenly blended.
3. Cover, and chill several hours to allow the flavors to meld.

Reduced Fat Yogurt Ranch Salad Dressing

Ingredients:

- 1 teaspoon dried parsley
- 1 teaspoon dried chives
- ½ teaspoon onion powder
- ¼ teaspoon ground black pepper
- ¼ teaspoon salt
- 2 cups lowfat plain yogurt
- ¼ cup powdered buttermilk
- 1 teaspoon garlic powder
- 1 teaspoon dried dill weed

Directions:

1. Combine buttermilk, garlic powder, dill weed, parsley, chives, onion powder, pepper, and salt in a bowl, making sure to break up any clumps.
2. Gently fold in the yogurt until combined, being careful not to over mix.
3. Refrigerate for 1 hour before serving. Pour off any whey before serving.
4. Serve immediately.

Sea Bass With Mango Chutney, Ginger, And Black Sesame Seeds

Ingredients:

Fat

- Two 6ounce striped bass fillets

- 1 tablespoon sesame oil

- Cooking spray

Other

- Salt and freshly milled black pepper to taste

- ¼ cup mango chutney

- 3 cups shredded iceberg lettuce

- 1 tablespoon minced fresh ginger (see note)

- 1 tablespoon soy sauce

- Ginger and Hot Red Pepper Vinaigrette

Directions:

1. Preheat the oven to 425°F. Spray an 8 X 8 X 8inch Pyrex baking dish with cooking spray.
2. Place the fillets in the baking dish. Sprinkle each fillet with ginger, soy sauce, and sesame oil. Lightly salt and pepper. Cover the dish with foil and bake for 10 minutes.
3. Remove from the oven and spoon 2 tablespoons of chutney onto each fillet. Return to the oven and bake, uncovered, for 5 more minutes.
4. Toss the shredded lettuce with the dressing. Divide between two plates and top each one with a fillet.

Roasted Butterfish

Ingredients:

Fat

- Four giant butterfish fillets

- 8 tablespoon butter or ghee

Other

- 4 cloves garlic

- 4 teaspoons freshly chopped thyme

- Pinch sea salt

- Juice from 1 lemon

Directions:

1. Begin by seasoning the butterfish fillets with a little bit of salt and place them on a plate.

2. Soften the butter, add the herbs and crushed garlic and blend all the pieces collectively in a small bowl.
3. Pour the butter combination over the fish.
4. Warm a nonstick pan over medium heat and add the fish.
5. Roast for about 2 to 3 minutes on both sides until cooked and the fish will get a crispy golden texture.
6. Be certain that the fillet is totally cooked by slicing into it. Cooked flesh will look opaque.
7. Place the fish onto a serving plate and squeeze a little bit of lemon over it. Serve sizzling.

www.ingramcontent.com/pod-product-compliance
Lightning Source LLC
Chambersburg PA
CBHW071456080526
44587CB00014B/2123